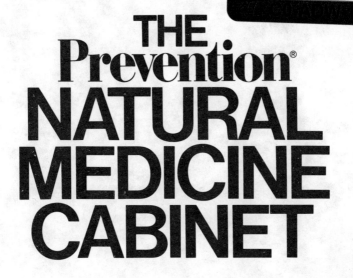

THE
Prevention®
NATURAL
MEDICINE
CABINET

by the editors of PREVENTION® magazine

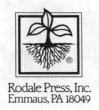

Rodale Press, Inc.
Emmaus, PA 18049

Contents

Introduction

Here's a quick reference guide to the everyday ailments that may trouble you and your family. With this booklet, you can quickly find natural remedies for the common maladies that probably send you to your medicine cabinet searching for relief.

With "The PREVENTION Natural Medicine Cabinet" you'll have effective, drug-free alternatives to laxatives, decongestants, aspirin, tranquilizers, sleeping pills, and more. You'll even find natural first aid for dealing with a poisoning. So keep this booklet handy for easy reference the next time you suffer from:

colds
sinus
coughs
joint pain
constipation
muscle aches
nervous tension
insomnia
cuts and abrasions
gas
diarrhea
hangover
and more!

And start taking advantage of the natural alternatives to drugs. □

NOTICE

The therapies discussed in this booklet are strictly adjunctive or complementary to medical treatment. Self-treatment can be hazardous with a serious ailment. We therefore urge you to seek out the best medical assistance you can find whenever it is needed.

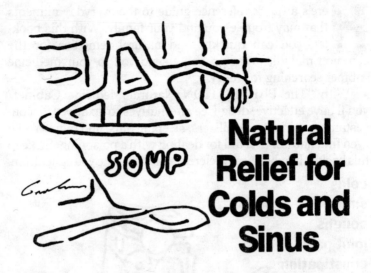

Natural Relief for Colds and Sinus

The same body machinery that causes stuffiness can help relieve it. Look to good habits, vitamins A and C, and super-soup.

Someone in the room sneezes. Germs fly out of his mouth at 100 miles an hour, swarming in the air. Inevitably, you breathe some of them in. Do they infect you? Not this time.

First, they're snared in a sticky layer of mucus. Then, cilia—tiny, hair-like stalks rooted in a second, deeper layer of mucus-secreting cells—sweep the top layer *and* the germs into your stomach. There, strong acids dispose of them—acids which, if it weren't for the protective layer of mucus in your stomach, would dispose of you, too.

Mucus. It's protected you since the time you were a gleam in your mother's eye. During ovulation, the mucus in the cervix turns thin and watery, helping sperm reach the uterus. After ovulation, it thickens, preventing germs from threatening what could be a developing fetus.

And mucus keeps on protecting.

Mucus from the salivary glands wraps food in a lubricating jacket that prevents you from choking.

Mucus in the digestive tract stops the absorption of useless or harmful materials.

And in the respiratory tract, mucus not only guards against infection, but also controls the temperature and humidity of inhaled air, and constantly clears away the tiny debris of dust and pollution.

How can one substance do all these things? Mucus is what scientists call semisolid, an elastic gel that changes depending on what it has to do. It can be sticky, soft, porous or water-resistant. But every mucus-producing cell in the body, no matter where it is, needs one substance to do its job right: vitamin A.

Without enough vitamin A, the mucous membranes would dry up. That happens in a *serious* deficiency. In a *slight* deficiency, the mucous membranes—particularly those of the respiratory tract—are weakened, and one symptom of such a deficiency is a cold.

Why a cold?

VULNERABLE TO VIRUSES

Remember, the mucus lining of the nose has two layers. If a lack of vitamin A weakens the top layer, a virus can penetrate it and infect the mucus-secreting cells below. (Scientists give these two layers one name: the mucosa.) Infected, the mucosa swells and pumps out thick mucus. And that thick mucus, while itself clogging up the nose, can also snag the top layer, stalling it. (Cilia normally move the top layer out of the nose every 10 minutes, making room for a new layer.) In short, you're all stuffed up.

But don't despair. Too little vitamin A may have gotten you into the problem (which is not unlikely, since a majority of adult Americans have a vitamin A deficiency), and a good dose of vitamin A could get you out.

Any stress—from a feverish cold to a car accident—robs the body of up to 60 percent of its vitamin A. "In such situations," writes Eli Seifter, Ph.D., a medical professor who has studied vitamin A, "large amounts of vitamin A are needed to replace the losses and to stimulate the immunologic responses weakened by the stress" (*Infectious Diseases,* September, 1975).

And one of those "immunologic responses," says Dr. Seifter, "is the ability of the mucosa to keep bacteria from inflaming already infected areas."

That means you need vitamin A to both protect *and* heal the mucosa. Vitamin A, too, is a natural alternative to decongestants, drugs that only make a cold *worse.*

"No clear-cut evidence exists for the efficacy of oral decongestants," writes a team of doctors in *Pediatrics* (April, 1975).

Spray decongestants, too, neither shrink the swollen mucosa nor clear mucus out of the nose.

What a spray decongestant actually does is to *temporarily* shrink the mucosa. But, if used repeatedly, it also chemically irritates it, and the mucosa swells up again later, becoming *more* swollen than before. Not only that, the decongestant lowers the amount of a natural antibiotic secreted by the mucosa, and partially cripples the cilia. The end result: congestion is worse. And, if you've used a spray decongestant, you could end up with a sinus infection.

A cold always infects the sinuses, those spaces above, behind and to the sides of your nose whose purpose scientists can't really explain. But that infection usually goes away with the cold. Spray decongestants, however, weaken the sinus mucosa, and may lead to sinusitis, a chronic sinus infection.

Spray decongestants aren't the only cause of sinusitis, of course. Just having a cold can start it. And anything that damages the cilia or slows the movement of the top layer of mucus—drinking alcohol, smoking cigarettes, breathing pollution or the dry air of some kinds of home heating—can set the stage for sinusitis.

But no matter what starts sinusitis, one symptom is always the same: postnasal drip, that steady flow of infected mucus down your throat. Other symptoms include a runny nose stuffed with yellow mucus, a poor sense of smell or hearing, and perhaps headaches.

How can you prevent sinusitis?

First, and most importantly, by getting enough vitamin A. Second, if you catch a cold, don't use decongestants. Third, blow your nose properly. Blowing your nose the wrong way can force infected mucus back into your sinuses, says Anthony J. Yonkers, M.D., an ear, nose and throat specialist from the University of Nebraska Medical Center. The right way to blow your nose is *gently*, without holding your nostrils shut.

Fourth, use a humidifier if your home heating system dries the air. The movement of the top mucus layer, which traps viruses and bacteria, is slowed by the dry air. When viruses and germs aren't moved quickly out of the nose, they're more likely to cause an infection.

And what if you get sinusitis?

Antibiotics aren't much help. A study shows that sinusitis patients who took antibiotics didn't recover any faster than patients not taking the drug (*Modern Medicine*, January 21, 1974).

HEAT CAN HELP

But there are natural treatments — that work. (And these remedies may work for any upper respiratory tract infection.)

"Heat, applied locally and in a warm, well-humidified room, promotes relief of pain and thinning of secretions," advises a team of doctors writing in the *Nebraska Medical Journal* (October, 1972).

And another doctor, Byron Baily, M.D., recommends applying that heat with hot towels — one to two hours four times a day (*American Family Physician*, December, 1973).

Drinking plenty of liquids — a time-honored remedy — also helps clear congestion. Double the amount you normally drink, using water, fruit juice and herbal teas. (Fenugreek, anise and sage teas are traditional herbal remedies for ridding yourself of mucus.)

And one liquid you shouldn't neglect is hot chicken soup.

A team of doctors at Mount Sinai Medical Center in Miami Beach, Florida, asked 15 healthy volunteers to drink hot chicken soup.

Before the volunteers drank the soup, the researchers measured their nasal mucus velocity — how fast the top layer of mucus moved out of the nose — and then measured it again after they drank the soup.

The researchers found that hot chicken soup increased nasal mucus velocity by 33 percent. When the volunteers drank cold water, nasal mucus velocity *decreased* by 28 percent.

"Hot rather than cold liquids might be preferable in the recommendations for fluid intake in patients with upper respiratory tract infections," they suggest (*Chest*, October, 1978).

But the "full prescription" for chicken soup, writes California physician Irwin Ziment, M.D., "also calls for the addition of plenty of pepper and garlic" (*Journal of the American Medical Association*, July 12, 1976).

Dr. Ziment points out that these spices are "expectorants," substances that thin mucus and clear it out of the system.

And although Dr. Ziment doesn't mention it, any list of expectorants should include not only garlic and cayenne pepper, but onion as well.

But sinusitis has another cause that none of these remedies can treat—nasal allergy. "Nasal allergy is an especially prominent predisposing factor [in sinusitis]," writes Dr. Bailey. For a nasal allergy, you need vitamin C.

A NATURAL ANTIHISTAMINE

The symptoms of nasal allergy—runny nose, inflamed and swollen mucosa—are caused by histamine, a chemical in the body. Vitamin C, studies show, is a natural *anti*-histamine.

Researchers had 17 healthy volunteers inhale histamine and measured their levels of "airway constriction." The next day, the volunteers again received histamine—but this time they got 500 milligrams of vitamin C first. With vitamin C, the degree of airway constriction was "significantly smaller" (*Journal of Allergy and Clinical Immunology*, April, 1973).

Since vitamin C could prevent the histamine-caused inflammation of the mucosa in nasal allergies, it could prevent and help treat sinusitis. The same goes for colds.

"If histamine plays a part in promoting mucosal inflammation in acute respiratory illness, the antihistamine action of vitamin C might explain, in part, the reduced symptoms and duration of these illnesses," writes a doctor commenting on a study in which vitamin C given to elementary school children with colds cut the length and severity of their infections (*New England Journal of Medicine*, March 14, 1974).

Mucus can be your friend or foe. Try making it your friend. □

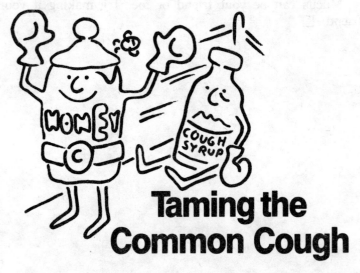

Taming the Common Cough

What's best for a nagging cough? Medical experts have nagging doubts about most over-the-counter remedies. But there are alternatives.

When spring arrives you can feel the breezes becoming warmer and gentler. People shake off the wintertime blahs and test new kites in the park. With the whole world about to burst into color, it would be a shame to be caught with a lingering cough from a February cold. But maybe you'll have one.

The question is: What to do about it?

When most people have a cough, they head for the nearest pharmacy and buy one of the many cough syrups, drops or capsules that are available without a prescription. In 1980, according to the U.S. Food and Drug Administration, Americans coughed up more than $1 billion for over-the-counter cough medications that claim to stop a cough outright or help clear the lungs of mucus.

But was that money well spent? Probably not. Since

1972, the FDA has been studying the effectiveness of cough medications, along with other nonprescription drugs, and has found that many don't live up to their advertised promises. Doctors often agree. One physician told us that over-the-counter cough medicines "aren't worth a darn, not any of them," and others say that natural remedies are safer, cost less and work just as well.

Sidney M. Wolfe, M.D., runs Public Citizen's Health Research Group, a Washington, D.C., consumer activist group that has sued the FDA to make that agency take ineffective drugs off the market faster, and has coauthored a book, *Pills That Don't Work* (Public Citizen's Health Research Group, 1980).

Based on research by Dr. Wolfe and others, here is a brief rundown of common cough-syrup ingredients, along with facts about their doubtful usefulness:

QUESTIONABLE INGREDIENTS

Expectorants. Manufacturers contend that these drugs increase the watery excretions produced by cells in the upper respiratory tract. Theoretically, those secretions loosen mucus and phlegm, making them easier to cough up and out of the lungs. But they often don't work as advertised.

"Expectorants are alleged to stimulate the flow of bronchial secretions," says one medical bulletin. "While there is no sound evidence to support this theory, these agents (terpin hydrate, ammonium chloride, guaifenesin, etc) are widely used" (*Harvard Medical School Health Letter*, November, 1978).

The FDA decided in 1976 that guaifenesin, which has been used in cough syrups since at least 1905, probably doesn't work. But so far, products containing this ingredient remain on the market, pending the outcome of lawsuits and laboratory tests.

While the expectorants probably don't work, that doesn't mean they're harmless. Large doses of aluminum chloride, for example, can upset the body's acid-base balance. Syrup of ipecac, another expectorant, may be toxic to young children and possibly adults, and terpin hydrate, mentioned before, may cause nausea and vomiting.

13

Even if expectorants *did* work, some cough medications don't contain enough. For example one popular bedtime cough remedy, which is 25 percent alcohol—*50 proof*—contains only about one-third the amount of expectorant said to be needed for effectiveness.

Suppressants. This group of medications tranquilizes or deactivates the part of the brain that controls the cough reflex. They shouldn't be used by anyone who has a "productive" cough, a cough that's doing its job of bringing up phlegm from the lungs.

"While it is tempting to interfere with Mother Nature's attempt to 'raise phlegm,' it is generally unwise to do so," says the *Harvard Medical School Health Letter.* "Such action will often prolong the siege and at worst may lead to serious breathing difficulties."

Suppressants shouldn't be given to people with coughs due to asthma or chronic bronchitis, the *Health Letter* points out. Those people rely on coughing to clear their lungs and, "giving large amounts of cough suppressants to such persons might lead to life-threatening results."

Antihistamines. Dr. Wolfe maintains that antihistamines thicken fluids in the lungs and make them more difficult to cough up—the opposite of the desired effect. He points out that one very popular cough syrup contains the antihistamine diphenhydramine as its only active ingredient, despite the fact that diphenhydramine hasn't been shown to stop coughs.

People who are kept awake at night with a cough due to postnasal "drip" sometimes use this kind of medication to dry their natural secretions, but that can be harmful. Dr. Wolfe says that antihistamines are appropriate only for allergies.

Decongestants. These drugs are not useful to anyone with a cough, says Brent Q. Hafen, Ph.D., in his book *The Self-Health Handbook* (Prentice-Hall, 1980). People with high blood pressure, diabetes, and heart or thyroid disease must avoid decongestants for health reasons, Dr. Hafen says, and most everyone else should do the same.

"Unless you are suffering from severe stuffiness and inability to breathe, you might be better off staying away from decongestants: They serve to dry up secretions and remove water from the system—exactly the opposite of what you need, which is to moisten and loosen the membranes," he says.

'SHOTGUN COMBINATIONS'

Multi-ingredient cough medicines. "Avoid the expensive, potentially harmful and essentially ineffective 'shotgun' cough-and-cold combinations," says Dr. Wolfe. These drugs, usually called "cold capsules," sometimes have conflicting effects on a cough.

"The various components [of a multi-ingredient medicine] may interact with one another to enhance toxicity, inhibit effectiveness or simply expose the consumer to extra unwanted side effects, often with no additional benefit," Dr. Wolfe writes.

Cough Drops. The American Dental Association points out that sugar is a hidden ingredient in many nonprescription drugs and that "some of the worst offenders are sugarladen cough drops and throat lozenges." This "medicinal candy," dentists say, causes cavities, especially when people carry boxes of "fruit-flavored cough drops, which attack their teeth all day long" (*American Pharmacy*, October, 1979).

Cough syrups are damaging too, because "their coating action not only soothes a cough but bathes the teeth in sugar long enough to trigger dental decay."

If you're shopping for cough syrups or drops, you'll find that they aren't equally sweet. One type of cough drop is 69 percent sugar, while another has no sugar. One company manufactures cough drops that contain 66.2, 22.0, 3.2, 2.5 and zero percent sugar. The sweetest cough syrup available contains 44 percent sugar, but others contain none.

If, despite the uncertainties, you do go shopping for an over-the-counter cough remedy, it might be a good idea to get some expert advice. Barbara Korberly, Pharm. D., of the Philadelphia College of Pharmacy and Science, says that pharmacists can't diagnose your problem, but they can give you valuable information about each medicine.

"People should go to their pharmacists and ask, 'What can I do for my cough?' The pharmacist may ask them, 'What is it that brings you here now? What is your major symptom?'"

The pharmacist will often be able to recommend to the consumer a remedy that will minimize his symptoms, will cause the fewest side effects, and will not conflict with the consumer's other medications or conditions, Dr. Korberly says.

15

DON'T OVERLOOK ALLERGY

Before a cough sufferer starts out for the pharmacy—if he does at all—he should try to get to the root of his cough. One often overlooked but highly treatable cause of a cough that outstays a cold is food allergy. Elmer Cranton, M.D., who specializes in preventive medicine and holistic therapies in Trout Dale, Virginia, says he has recognized a "postflu milk-allergy syndrome."

"A cough that hangs on after a cold is commonly an unsuspected food allergy," says Dr. Cranton. "Someone might have been eating a lot of a certain food they were sensitive to, usually milk or wheat or a combination of foods, but didn't know it. And there were no symptoms of an allergy until after they caught a cold or the flu."

To discover the guilty food, Dr. Cranton proceeds with an elimination diet—all suspect foods are removed from the diet for seven to 10 days, then are reintroduced to the patient one by one until something provokes an allergic response. Dairy products, wheat products, yeast, eggs and citrus are common allergens, he says.

"We've found that only six or seven days after elimination of the offender, the cough stops. Afterwards, if they stay away from that food for a month or so, they can frequently begin eating it and slowly build up their tolerance to it again."

Other physicians have also found a link between coughing and allergy. Ernest K. Cotton, M.D., a lung expert at the University of Colorado Health Sciences Center in Denver, says that "allergic skin testing may be important in some patients," and a British specialist says that "most recurrent coughs, if not due to colds, are allergic in origin" (*British Medical Journal*, August, 1976).

Regarding over-the-counter cough medications, Dr. Cranton says, "I tell my patients to use as little of them as they can get away with," because they might mask a serious illness and because they contain suspicious chemicals.

"Nobody's tested them in combination," he continues. "Each one by itself might be harmless, but when you look at all of them together, they might do some harm.

"I think that one of the reasons we're seeing more and more allergies to good foods like milk and wheat, is the great burden of foreign substances we're exposed to—in over-the-counter drugs, food additives and pollution. The average American consumes five to six pounds of chemicals a year," he says.

HOME REMEDIES THAT WORK

Dr. Cranton and many other physicians say that simple home remedies are sometimes best for coughs. He recommends putting a dab of honey (in moderation) on the back of the tongue. And he believes that good nutrition, with emphasis on small amounts of selenium and vitamins C and E, "increases the tolerance to colds and coughs by maintaining the integrity of the organism."

For a postnasal-drip-related cough that might keep you from sleeping, one source advises sleeping on your stomach.

Lots of fluids, such as fruit juices and chicken soup, work better than expectorants, others say. Vaporizers and humidifiers sometimes help a cough, but adding aromatic jellies to the steam may lower the body's resistance to infection, according to Dr. Hafen.

At any rate, most normal, uncomplicated coughing, as one British authority put it, is "a necessary evil" and resolves by itself. And Dr. Wolfe says, "Coughing, especially if you are coughing something up, is a healthy way to clear your respiratory tract. If a cough lasts more than a week or if you are having difficulty breathing . . . consult a nurse or doctor." □

Put the Freeze on Pain

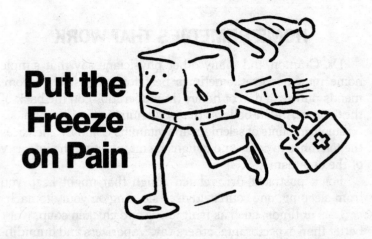

There's a pain-relief giant lurking in your kitchen freezer. Here's how to make him work for you.

The iceman cometh. That may not sound like good news to those who've been out battling the ravages of Old Man Winter. But if you're suffering from a toothache, a sprain, bursitis, rheumatoid arthritis or any one of a host of other painful afflictions, it could be welcome news indeed because ice can be a healing helper.

The modern medical term is *cryotherapy*, or *cold therapy*, but the idea of ice therapy has probably been around ever since some Ice Age human with a badly sprained ankle hobbled across a glacial stream and noticed the cold water had a numbing effect on the pain. Over the centuries cold therapy became an important remedy to kill the pain and reduce the swelling of sprains and fractures, to cool a fever or to soothe a headache. Medical science and modern refrigeration methods have only expanded its uses, and new reports of the therapeutic value of cold therapy keep coming in all the time.

18

Take the study conducted by doctors and physical therapists at Germantown Medical Center in Philadelphia. The four-week trial involved 24 rheumatoid arthritis patients with painful knees. The patients were asked simply to place an ice pack (six ice cubes and a quart of water in a plastic bag) above and below one knee for 20 minutes, three times a day. The other knee wasn't iced, so that the patients could judge the effectiveness of the treatment. The results were assessed by various tests and by a visual pain-rating scale.

After the "baggietherapy," as the researchers called their treatment, "there was statistically significant improvement in knee range-of-motion, strength, timed functional tests, and the sleep duration of patients, as well as a decrease in ... pain scale and oral analgesic intake" (*Journal of the American Medical Association*, July 24, 1981).

"The use of cryotherapy represents a major analgesic [painkiller] in rheumatoid arthritis," concluded Peter D. Utsinger, M.D., who directed the study. The ice-bag treatment "is an acceptable substitute for oral analgesics, is associated with increased functional status, is unassociated with obvious side effects, is inexpensive, and does not appear to mediate its effect by altering protein or cellular constituents of synovial fluid."

In other words, a plastic bag full of ice cubes on the knee can be as good as aspirin down the hatch. Better really, when you consider that the ice treatment has none of the dangers associated with long-term aspirin use.

THE BODY HEALS ITSELF

But that's only the tip of the ice bag. The beauty of cold therapy is that, besides being inexpensive and simple to use, it doesn't interfere with the body's own healing processes. And it can be used in combination with other forms of treatment, which is why many hospital emergency rooms, postoperative recovery rooms and physical-therapy departments have their own ice-making machines on the premises.

"We generally ice any presentation of acute pain," says Rebecca Deweese, senior physical therapist on the staff of West Virginia University Medical Center.

Ms. Deweese told us that many physical therapists use a

combination of ice and compression to control the swelling of injured and inflamed joints. An Ace bandage is wrapped around the affected area — say an ankle — and then an ice pack is placed on it. The area is kept elevated to drain fluid away from it. "Ice in combination with compression is generally better than either treatment used alone to reduce swelling," says Ms. Deweese.

You can now buy for home use a special cold compression wrap, consisting of a reusable gel pack that is cooled in your kitchen freezer, and an Ace bandage with a pocket in it to keep the cold pack in place. One advantage of the device is that it allows mobility while maintaining cold directly on the injury. It's a convenient form of first-aid treatment for muscle strains and spasms, sprains, tendinitis simple headaches, and insect bites.

COLD WITHOUT ICE

You can even take your cold therapy far from mechanical sources of refrigeration, with a product that creates cold by a chemical reaction inside a sealed plastic bag. Although the chemical compress can be used only once, it might become a handy addition to the first-aid kits of campers and hikers, especially those headed into snake-infested country. Once recent report indicates that immediate treatment with ice packs or instant cold packs reduces the extent of injury and time of hospitalization for victims of poisonous snake bites (*New England Journal of Medicine*, October 29, 1981).

Chances are you won't be running into any poisonous snakes in the near future, but there's another kind of "bite" that most people have experienced at one time or another: the kind your own teeth give you when you have a cavity. And once again, ice can help.

Of course, you can just hold an ice bag against your jaw, but some Canadian researchers have found a new way of treating dental pain that involves a combination of ice massage and acupuncture. They've successfully taught a number of dental clinic patients to lessen the discomfort of toothache.

To show just how effective the technique is, researchers conducted an experiment involving 40 patients at the outpatient dental clinic of Montreal General Hospital. Some of the patients were taught to gently massage with a piece of ice a particular acupuncture point of the hand on the same side as the pain. The point lies in the fleshy web between the thumb and index finger. It was already known that acupuncture applied to this point could relieve dental pain. As a control, other patients massaged the point, but with a wooden ball instead of ice. A pain questionnaire was administered to both groups to measure the degree of pain relief.

Even though both groups showed similar levels of pain before the experiment, pain reduction was significantly greater among the patients who massaged with ice. Ice massage decreased the intensity of pain by 50 percent or more in the majority of patients treated (*Canadian Medical Association Journal*, January 26, 1980).

"We don't know the exact mechanism involved," one of the researchers, Ronald Melzack, Ph.D., told us. "The theory is that ice massage of the point activates areas of the brain stem—the periaquaductal area—that are known to inhibit pain signals." Dr. Melzack has also conducted a study that indicates ice massage of other acupuncture points can alleviate low back pain and other forms of chronic pain.

Cold therapy has many internal applications as well. One doctor uses it to treat ulcers and control food cravings in his patients.

CHILLING THE APPETITE

"Drinking a glass of ice water has a shrinking effect on the stomach," says Richard A. Hansen, M.D. "It suppresses the appetite and makes you feel full. Which is why some restaurants serve ice water before meals. It lets them serve smaller portions and still make their customers feel satisfied after the meal. At home you'd be reaching for seconds."

Ice water also decreases stomach acidity, according to Dr. Hansen, who is director of the Poland Spring Health Institute in Maine. "A glass of ice water—especially a neutral pH mineral water—is a lot better for an ulcer patient than a glass of milk, which actually stimulates the secretion of stomach acid," he says.

Dr. Hansen cautions people with diabetes and circulatory diseases such as arteriosclerosis, as well as older people with poor circulation, to use ice packs or cold drinks only under a doctor's supervision. There are other, more rare circumstances when cold therapy shouldn't be used at all, as in cases of Raynaud's phenomenon, certain collagen and blood diseases, and when a patient is hypersensitive to cold.

For most people, though, it's difficult to think of a safer method of pain relief than a bag of ice cubes.

"Ice packs can be used intermittently—one hour on, 10 minutes off—for hours at a time on areas like the shoulder, where circulation is good," says Dr. Hansen. For areas like the foot and hand, the ice bag should be wrapped in a towel.

Following these simple rules, you can go a long way toward eliminating the soreness of everyday aches and pains without having to resort to expensive and possibly harmful pain-killing drugs.

Just remember this the next time you have an ache: Leave the aspirin bottle in the medicine cabinet, reach for the ice-cube tray instead, and send that pain to Siberia. □

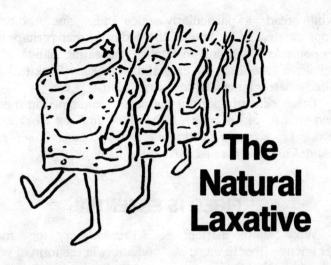

The Natural Laxative

Your 'gut reaction' to bran shows why it can protect you against many common diseases.

"**A** dog, fed on fine white bread and water ... does not live beyond the 50th day. A dog fed on the coarse (whole wheat) bread of the military, lives and keeps his health."

The results of a recent scientific investigation into the merits of whole wheat versus white bread? Hardly. It is the report of an experiment done by a French physiologist, recorded in the British medical journal *Lancet* of March 11, 1826!

Nevertheless, 99 years later, Morris Fishbein, M.D., former editor of the *Journal of the American Medical Association*, could write that the "standard white bread loaf, that forms the large portion of bread baked in the United States today, is the product to be recommended as most satisfactory."

Since as early as Greek and Roman times, the controversy has raged over refined white flour versus unrefined brown flour with the bran, or outer husk of the wheat, not milled away.

Brown bread was the food of peasants and simple country folk. White bread was for the wealthy city folks with supposedly sophisticated palates.

By the end of the 18th century, the trend toward eating

white bread was particularly evident in England. And so it is appropriate, and a bit ironic, that today the man perhaps most responsible for trying to change the eating habits of the "civilized" world is an Englishman—Denis Burkitt, M.D., affectionately known as the "Bran Man."

Dr. Burkitt's important message is contained in the title and subtitle of his book, *Eat Right—To Keep Healthy and Enjoy Life More: How Simple Diet Changes Can Prevent Many Common Diseases* (Arco Publishing, 1979).

FIBER IS ESSENTIAL

What "simple diet changes"? Primarily, making sure we get enough fiber in our diets, preferably in the form of whole wheat bread and miller's (unprocessed) wheat bran.

What "common diseases"? Although it may sound incredible, Dr. Burkitt says that eating about two heaping tablespoons of miller's bran every day can help prevent constipation, diverticulosis, appendicitis, hiatal hernia, varicose veins, hemorrhoids, colon cancer, diabetes and even obesity. Today, many other researchers are investigating the effects of fiber and bran in our diets and confirming the benefits observed by Dr. Burkitt.

How does such humble stuff as bran perform its seeming miracles? Basically by keeping our bowel movements "regular" and by decreasing their "transit time"—that is, the time it takes for stools to move through and out of the colon (large intestine).

Although bran is sometimes called "roughage," Dr. Burkitt likes to call it "softage" because it has a softening effect on hard stools, thus relieving constipation. On the other hand, if you have diarrhea, bran can relieve that as well. How is that possible? Because bran normalizes bowel functions and makes stools easy to pass.

"When diets are rich in dietary fiber," says Dr. Burkitt, "stools passed are usually large in volume, pale in color, soft in consistency, and float in water. The reverse is true of fiber-depleted diets." Interestingly, bran is now even being given to surgical patients before their operations to help make certain their bowels are not clogged after the operations.

WIDE-RANGE PROTECTION

Now, let's look at some of the common diseases that bran can help protect you against, and see if you don't agree that the very same bran we used to throw away or feed to animals is a remarkable, necessary part of our daily diets.

• Diverticular disease. Also called diverticulosis, this disease is the development of small, blown-out pouches in the colon. When one of these pouches, or diverticula, becomes inflamed, the stabbing pain lets us know it.

"In Western countries," says Dr. Burkitt, "about one in 10 people over the age of 40 and one in three over 60 have diverticular disease. Constipation is now recognized as the underlying cause."

According to Dr. Burkitt and others, hard stools are what causes the problem in the first place. It just takes too much effort or pressure for your colon to push along the hard feces, and the result is one or more outpouchings. To prevent the disease in the first place, you need to eat the same bran you'd eat to prevent constipation. But what if you *already* have diverticulosis?

Remarkably, doctors used to prescribe a *low*-fiber diet for those who already had diverticular disease. Now just the opposite is true.

"In almost all British clinics and in an increasing proportion of American clinics, all patients with diverticular disease of the colon, whether with or without symptoms, are put on high-fiber diets," says Dr. Burkitt. "In some hospitals this approach has reduced the proportion of patients requiring surgical treatment by as much as 90 percent."

• Appendicitis. Appendicitis? Can an inflammation like appendicitis be caused by eating too little fiber? Yes, indeed.

According to Dr. Burkitt, the appendix is often first blocked by a "small hard lump of fecal matter, about the size of a pea ... This exists only in the presence of the firmer feces that are associated with fiber-depleted diets." Once blocked, the appendix becomes infected.

"Keeping the bowel content soft seems to provide the best safe-guard against the development of appendicitis," says Dr. Burkitt. "Sufficient fiber in the diet will do this."

RELIEVING THE STRAIN

• Hiatal hernia, varicose veins and hemorrhoids. According to Dr. Burkitt, each of these conditions is probably caused by constipation and the resulting straining at stool. As you strain, you raise tremendously the pressure in your abdominal cavity. Over a period of time, such constant straining and raised pressure can have several undesirable effects.

First, the increased pressure can cause the top of your stomach to push through your diaphragm, which in medical jargon is called a hiatal hernia.

Second, when you strain at stool, you actually force the blood in your leg veins to flow backward. Over a period of time, this backward flow stretches the veins, weakening the action of the small valves in the leg veins that prevent this backward flow. The result: swollen, painful varicose veins.

Third, "until recently it has always been assumed that piles (hemorrhoids) are varicosities of the veins in the anal canal analogous to varicose veins in the legs," says Dr. Burkitt, "but recent research has suggested that this is not in fact the case. It now seems that piles are a downward prolapse (protrusion) of normal (anal) cushions full of blood vessels that surround the upper end of the anal canal to help prevent the escape of feces. These cushions are present from birth. When they are swollen and are pushed down through the anal canal they are called piles ... When the stool is hard, the straining that is necessary for evacuation forces blood into the cushions, which swell up as a result ... A diet rich in fiber is the best way to guard against a recurrence of the problem."

• Colon cancer. While admittedly a hotly debated issue, "it is currently agreed," says Dr. Burkitt, "that dietary changes are likely to be dominant in the causation of colorectal cancer. Both increased fat and diminished fiber intake are characteristic of high-risk communities."

Eating fat causes an increased production of bile acids by the liver, and Dr. Burkitt believes that changes in fecal bacteria may be responsible for turning the normally harmless bile acids into potentially carcinogenic (cancer-causing) substances. Eating bran has the advantage both of creating large volume stools, which may dilute the carcinogens, and of decreasing transit time so that the carcinogens will be in contact with the gut for less time.

Two recent animal studies have shown the effect of fiber on colon cancer. In one case, colon tumors were significantly reduced as fiber intake increased; in the other, colon tumors were also greatly reduced as bran intake went up and fat intake went down (*Canadian Journal of Surgery*, January, 1980; *Journal of the National Cancer Institute*, April, 1979).

A CHANGE FOR DIABETICS

• Diabetes. "It has been customary," says Dr. Burkitt, "to advise diabetic patients to take a little sugar and to reduce starch; this leaves a diet containing a larger proportion of fat. Recently many diabetic experts have begun to advise patients to take more starch and less fat as part of their special diet."

Dr. Burkitt points out that the trends are now changing for the better as more doctors recommend unrefined, high-fiber starch foods such as whole wheat bread. "In the United States," says Dr. Burkitt, "papers have been published in medical journals reporting that a diet of unrefined high-fiber starch (constituting 60 percent of daily calorie intake with sugar reduced to five percent, fat to 20 percent and protein left at 15 percent) caused a remission of the disease in 85 percent of the patients. These diets contain much dietary fiber — about two ounces (70 grams) daily."

And as researchers at the University of Kentucky School of Medicine have put it, high-carbohydrate diets that are rich in fiber "may be the treatment of choice" for patients with mild to moderate diabetes (*Cereal Foods World*, August, 1976).

• Obesity. What could too much body fat possibly have to do with too little plant fiber? Plenty, according to the Bran Man.

First, fiber itself contains no calories — the only food in our diet with that distinction.

Second, people tend to eat less of whole wheat bread or cake or biscuits than of those made from refined white flour. "Bulky high-fiber foods ... fill you up and consequently fewer calories are consumed," says Dr. Burkitt. And contrary to popular belief, high-fiber foods are not "fattening" for the very reason that they do contain a lot of fiber.

27

Bran also seems to help us actually get rid of calories. In a recent study done on the effect of wheat bran on the calories we take in, researchers at Oregon State University discovered that their subjects lost 18 percent more calories through their stools when they consumed a half-ounce of wheat bran per day than when they did not (*American Journal of Clinical Nutrition*, June, 1979).

Dr. Burkitt is the first to admit that his observations do not mean that "fiber-depleted diets are the only cause of the diseases mentioned, but merely one of many. The destruction of the single span of a multispan bridge crossing a river will suffice to impede the progress of an invading army. Likewise, the removal of one of several causes of a disease may be sufficient to greatly reduce its prevalence. If fiber deficiency is one cause . . . it is probably the most easily assailable of all causative factors.

"This epitomizes the commonsense approach. Had the farmer postponed his sowing until he understood the process of seed germination, he would have died of starvation." □

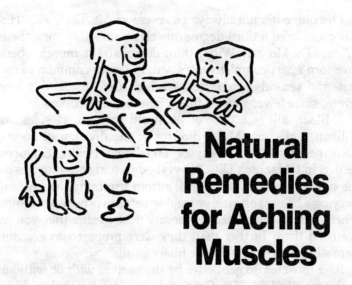

Natural Remedies for Aching Muscles

A strained muscle can mean days of pain and inconvenience. Now you can shorten your recovery time with these self-care remedies.

M r. Packer looked and felt young for his age so he automatically said "yes" when his son asked for his help moving an old refrigerator. Besides, they had the use of a dolly to support most of the weight.

The move went very smoothly, too, until they tried to get the refrigerator off the dolly. Mr. Packer's biceps just couldn't quite handle the load. Suddenly there was a snapping sound and a sharp pain. Mr. Packer's arm became very weak and there was a lump the size of a golf ball where his muscle was supposed to be.

"This is a common injury," says Stephen Morgan, D.O., of the Sports Medicine Clinic in Traverse City, Michigan, and the doctor who treated Mr. Packer.

"We see injuries like this all the time, and it's usually someone who overestimates his or her own muscular capabilities. The next thing you know they've strained an arm, calf, groin or hamstring muscle.

Of course it's not always as severe as Mr. Packer's. "His was considered a third-degree muscle strain—the worst there is," says Dr. Morgan. With a third-degree strain, muscle fibers have torn apart completely. It's actually more common to see first- and second-degree strains, which are considerably less severe, since fewer muscle fibers have been disrupted.

"Milder still is a case of plain old sore muscles," adds William A. Grana, M.D., director of the division of sports medicine at the University of Oklahoma Health Sciences Center, in Oklahoma City. "Everybody's had sore muscles at one time or another, whether it's from trimming the hedges, carrying a heavy suitcase, or jogging before a proper warm-up. When your muscles become sore it just means that you've stretched them further than they were prepared to go. But there's been no tearing of the fibers at all."

Sore muscles do get better by themselves with or without treatment. "In fact," Dr. Grana told us, "most muscle strains do, too. But you can aid the process dramatically with some simple home remedies."

"Immediately after the injury and for the first 24 to 48 hours, I recommend RICE," says Dr. Morgan. And he doesn't mean the kind you eat, either. This kind of RICE is actually an acronym for Rest, Ice, Compression and Elevation.

"Rest means to stop whatever you're doing," says Frank Bassett III, M.D., professor of orthopedic surgery at Duke University Medical Center, in Durham, North Carolina. "Usually, that's an automatic response because of the severe pain that hits at the moment the injury occurs.

"Interestingly enough," says Dr. Bassett, "the pain experienced from a muscle strain is only partly due to the tearing of the muscle fibers. At least half of what you feel (or more) is due to the muscle spasms that accompany the injury."

In a spasm, the muscles surrounding the injured part vigorously contract and hold that position—sometimes for days. These spasms, while intensely painful, are actually the body's way of protecting itself from further injury. That's because a contracted muscle acts like a built-in splint, immobilizing the damaged part in much the same way a cast immobilizes a broken leg.

If you're lucky enough not to be in extreme pain, don't take that as a license to continue using that muscle, advises Dr.

Morgan. Once the fibers have torn even a little, as in a first-degree muscle strain, overdoing it can lead to a second — or even third-degree injury.

As soon as possible after you've strained or pulled a muscle, get ice onto it. "Ice is extremely important in muscle strains because of its ability to stop the internal bleeding and reduce the swelling," explains Dr. Grana.

AVOIDING SCAR TISSUE

Dr. Morgan agrees. "When muscle fibers tear it causes some bleeding and swelling. Ice constricts the blood vessels and stops the bleeding, which in turn counters the painful swelling. That's important because if the bleeding continues it causes an influx of white blood cells to the injury site. Ordinarily you'd want those cells to come because they are the ones that fight infection. In a muscle injury, however, there aren't any germs to fight, yet that doesn't stop the white blood cells from going about their business anyway. And that includes releasing enzymes that destroy dead muscle tissue.

"So the more bleeding you have, the more tissue destruction you have. And once muscle tissue is destroyed, it's replaced with scar tissue. And that's bad," explains Dr. Morgan, "because scar tissue does not have the ability to contract like normal, healthy muscle. It's fibrous material that just sits there and doesn't do anything.

"Ice also helps reduce pain because it has a numbing effect," adds Dr. Bassett. "But be careful how you apply it. Ice in direct contact with your skin can cause a cold burn or blister. Instead put the ice in a plastic bag and then wrap a towel around the whole thing. Always be sure there is a cloth between the ice and your skin."

If you don't have any ice cubes available, be innovative. A cold can of orange juice or even a frozen leg of lamb can serve the same purpose as a bag of ice cubes.

Dr. Bassett recommends applying the cold for 10 to 15 minutes at a time, three or four times a day.

Dr. Morgan suggests doing it every two hours for 20 minutes. And all agree that ice therapy should continue for 24 to 48 hours.

A SNUG WRAP

Compression, the third component of RICE, should also be continued for that period, but only if there's swelling. Wrap the injured muscle with an elastic bandage snugly but not so tight it impedes circulation. To be sure that's not happening, unwrap the area when you remove the ice and check to be sure that all is still rosy.

Elevation, the last part of the self-treatment program, gets gravity working for you instead of against you. Of course, some muscles lend themselves to elevation more easily than others, so adjust accordingly.

By now you may be wondering why you've been keeping a heating pad in the closet all these years. Wasn't it heat that made your pulled muscles feel good? Is it now considered a mistake to use heat?

According to the doctors we spoke to, the answer to these questions is—what else?—yes *and* no.

"The only time heat is an acceptable therapy," says Dr. Morgan, "is when the muscles are simply sore, not strained. If there's any swelling or discoloration, then you've strained the muscle to some degree. If there's no swelling then it's probably only a sore muscle, nothing more, and applying heat will not only feel good but may increase flexibility.

"There's a lot of gray area involved in diagnosing a muscle strain. A good gauge, besides swelling, is pain. Usually, the more it hurts, the more it's injured. When there's been a rupture of the muscle fibers, heat would only *increase* the bleeding, swelling and pain—delaying your recovery time.

"Some doctors recommend heat therapy once the bleeding and swelling have gone down—usually after about 48 hours of ice therapy. But I won't even use heat on recovering muscles. I just don't think it's worth the chance of restarting the bleeding. Even professional football teams use only ice in their treatment of strained muscles."

HEAT FOR REHABILITATION

Drs. Bassett and Grana agree, but only in part. They both believe that heat treatment serves a purpose in the rehabilitation stage of strained muscles.

Once the muscle is on the road to recovery—that is, the pain and swelling are down—applying heat will increase the blood flow, bringing in nutrients and cells that speed the healing process.

"What's more," says Dr. Grana, "heat improves the muscle's elasticity and helps get back its range of motion."

To warm up a hurt muscle you can use an electric heating pad or hot-water bottle. If you don't have one handy, soak a towel in warm water, wrap it around the injured muscle and then cover it with several layers of plastic wrap. This will hold in the heat and help prevent dripping.

You may also want to try one of the over-the-counter cream rubs advertised to promote local heating. "These rubs dilate blood vessels in the skin," says Dr. Morgan. "This creates a warming effect, which makes the sore muscle feel more comfortable."

"Using these rubs during the time of recovery can also help improve mobility and flexibility," Dr. Bassett adds. "The important thing is not to use heat therapy too soon. Let your symptoms be the guide. And remember, if you've still got a lot of swelling and pain after a couple of days, it's time to see a doctor. You could be dealing with a much more serious injury, such as torn ligaments or broken bones."

Once your hurt muscles have begun to heal, you should begin some gentle exercising, gradually increasing the load. The object is to strengthen the muscle that was strained so it will be better able to resist reinjury.

In fact, with the proper care you can prevent muscle strains from happening in the first place, according to the doctors we spoke to. "Most strains occur when you are fatigued or caught off balance," Dr. Bassett told us. "So use your common sense." Don't plan a tennis game after cleaning out the attic, for example.

"Stretching exercises done before a particularly strenuous task can help prevent a muscle pull also," says Dr. Morgan. "Just before a long walk or yard work, stretch the muscles you'll be using.

"It's the most important preventive measure there is." □

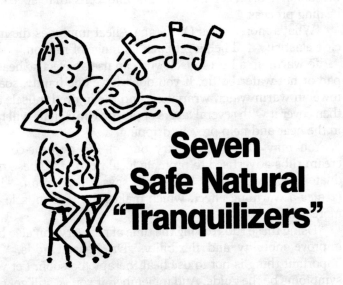

Seven Safe Natural "Tranquilizers"

When your nerves are shot, consider your possible need for vitamins, minerals and other safe ways to keep your cool.

Millie's a nervous wreck. The holidays are fast approaching and she's got so much left to do. Company's coming and the house is a mess. The spare room really could use a coat of paint and new curtains. And what about food? She wants it to be special, but when will she find time to prepare it all? Then there are gifts to buy and wrap, and, after all, the kids and her husband still need clean clothes for school and work.

It's not that her family isn't understanding. They try to help, but she finds herself snapping at them anyway, or even screaming for silly, foolish reasons. Later she feels so guilty about it. Yet she can't seem to help herself.

Millie's doctor assures her that there's nothing seriously wrong with her. Her irritability, nervousness and anxiety are probably temporary, and perhaps a tranquilizer will help ease her over the rough spots.

If Millie decides to take the prescription, she certainly won't be alone. Some doctors say that many people who take tranquilizing drugs are on the wrong track. The right track, they say, can be as simple as changing your eating habits.

A case of "nerves" can often be triggered by nutrient deficiencies resulting from a poor diet. On top of that, anxiety and stressful situations of any kind often increase the need for certain vitamins and minerals, compounding the problem. In other words, the difference between Millie and a "normal" person isn't that Millie has a *tranquilizer* deficiency, she has a *nutrient* deficiency. Her body's own natural "tranquilizers" have been depleted.

NIACIN IS EFFECTIVE

Fact is, Millie would be much better off trying a safe alternative such as niacin. This concept is not new. Niacin, also called nicotinamide, has been used successfully as a tranquilizer for more than 20 years in certain psychiatric circles. But it had the misfortune of being introduced at about the same time as the tranquilizer Valium, only minus the fanfare.

"Niacin was an orphan drug, belonging to everyone because it was in the public domain," wrote Humphry Osmond, M.D., and Abram Hoffer, M.D., Ph.D., noted authorities on orthomolecular psychiatry. "Consequently it was in no one's interest to promote it by advertising or to advance it politically" (*Journal of Orthomolecular Psychiatry,* vol. 9, no. 3, 1980).

Apparently, that is no longer the case. A researcher group from the Hoffman-La Roche company of Switzerland compares the vitamin's effectiveness to that of the minor tranquilizers.

According to H.L. Newbold, M.D., author of *Mega-Nutrients for Your Nerves* (Peter H. Wyden, 1975), "while most people feel better within days of beginning a niacin regimen, some require months to feel the benefits. It is especially important to give this vitamin a lengthy therapeutic trial because its potential benefits are so great."

Michael Lesser, M.D., author of *Nutrition and Vitamin Therapy* (Grove Press, 1980), agrees. "In using niacin, I begin with a modest dose of 50 mg. three times a day and build up to the optimal level, the dose that achieves maximum improvement."

35

However, "needs vary from person to person and even from day to day," add E. Cheraskin, M.D., D.M.D., and W.M. Ringsdorf Jr., D.M.D., of the department of oral medicine at the University of Alabama in Birmingham. "The only surefire way to overcome or avoid depletion is to consume daily doses of nutrients severalfold the levels specified as 'recommended daily allowances.'"

"Niacin, like other nutrients, should be taken with meals, as vitamins work together with the food," says Dr. Lesser. And while you're at it, eat foods rich in niacin, such as lean meats (not pork), poultry, fish, peanuts, brewer's yeast, wheat germ and liver.

RELIEVING PREMENSTRUAL TENSION

Millie might feel even better if she also adds vitamin B6 (pyridoxine) to her regimen about a week to 10 days before each menstrual period. That's when premenstrual tension normally strikes her (and about 80 percent of all other menstruating women).

Yet B6 taken prior to menstruating could virtually eliminate the discomfort for most of them. That's what studies seem to suggest.

In one recent experiment, conducted by Joel T. Hargrove, M.D., and Guy E. Abraham, M.D., 25 women suffering from moderate to severe premenstrual tension first either received vitamin B6 or a placebo (a look-alike, nontherapeutic pill) for three consecutive menstrual cycles, followed by the other treatment during the next three cycles. Of the 25 patients, 21 showed a significant decrease in their symptoms while taking the B6 but not while they were using the placebo (Infertility, vol. 3, 1980).

Some doctors believe that high estrogen levels after ovulation may play some part in either an increased need for, or a lower ability to absorb, vitamin B6, and the resulting deficiency leads to premenstrual tension.

But it isn't only women who feel when B6 levels go down. A deficiency can make anyone irritable, tired or restless.

When you begin taking B6, says Dr. Newbold, you may find that you have more energy and feel less tense. Some people find that B6 actually relaxes them to the point of sleepiness, and if this is the case, take your dose at bedtime.

Some doctors recommend beginning with a daily dose of 50 mg., which is almost always enough to relieve tension. Of course, people are different, and what works best for one may not be be the first choice for another. So if the B vitamins aren't a hit with you, maybe your case of "nerves" will respond to vitamin C.

"The influence of vitamin C on the mental state is quite remarkable," notes Dr. Lesser.

Even though vitamin C cannot be made in the brain, concentration there is higher than any other organ except the adrenal glands. "It should not be surprising that it plays a major role in brain function," explain Drs. Osmond and Hoffer. "The body would not make an effort to maintain a high level in the brain when for most people the whole body contains just enough to prevent scurvy but not enough for optimum health."

In fact, Drs. Osmond and Hoffer think that vitamin C may be a "naturally occurring antianxiety substance." This makes sense, especially when you consider that scurvy is characterized by severe tension and sometimes psychosis.

"We have seen several schizophrenic patients who responded to 10 grams per day of ascorbic acid (vitamin C) with marked relief from anxiety and tension, when no tranquilizer had been helpful," notes Drs. Osmond and Hoffer.

Remember, that's for very sick people. Dr. Lesser says that "vitamin C in doses of one or two grams at a time works as a tranquilizer for the anxious."

So do calcium and magnesium, according to many other specialists.

CALMING NERVES WITH CALCIUM

"Calcium deficiencies generally sneak up slowly," warn Drs. Cheraskin and Ringsdorf, who are also the authors of *Psycho-dietetics: Food as the Key to Emotional Health* (Stein and Day, 1974). "Normally the body protects itself from blood-level fluctuations by drawing upon bone and muscle reserves. But the nervous system cannot continue 'stealing' calcium indefinitely," explain the doctors. "Eventually the balance must be restored with calcium-rich foods. A tiny decrease of calcium in the blood can produce uncontrollable temper outbursts."

Yet that can happen, especially during times of sudden, unexpected emotional stress. That's because at those times the blood lactic-acid levels can rise considerably, which has the effect of depleting circulating calcium. The result is a case of "nerves" or a volatile temper.

Calcium alone has been used with great success, but calcium along with magnesium or even magnesium alone also exert "tranquilizing" effects.

August F. Daro, M.D., has seen for himself just how well the two minerals work. Dr. Daro, professor emeritus of obstetrics and gynecology at Stritch School of Medicine in Maywood, Illinois, often uses magnesium with calcium or magnesium by itself as a tranquilizer for patients who complain of nervousness or insomnia.

"Some people drink a lot of soft drinks and coffee, or they use diuretics, all of which rob the body of vital minerals," says Dr. Daro. "Then they come in and complain of nervousness. They want something to quiet their nerves. I give them magnesium and calcium. It's not habit-forming. They feel quite good afterwards. It's amazing to see how these patients are so very happy, how much calmer than they were before."

Vitamins and minerals can do wonders for your nerves, but so can vigorous physical exercise. That's what researchers from Stanford University School of Medicine discovered recently. They tested 81 previously sedentary middle-aged men for a one-year period. Those selected randomly to run on a regular basis during the year showed significantly less anxiety than the control group (*Internal Medicine News,* June 1, 1981).

SOOTHING SELECTIONS

If you're not up for a workout like that, then drop into an easy chair and turn on some music. Researchers have found that music can help to relax tense muscles, promote rest and relieve troubled moods.

Musical selections aimed at inducing relaxation should have a steady, reassuring rhythm, low-frequency tones, soothing orchestral effects and a comforting, serene melody (*CMA Journal,* November 4, 1978).

Since the therapeutic effects of music are closely tied to personal associations and memories, don't be overinfluenced by the recommendations of others, no matter how well intended. Choose music that has special meaning for you, and experiment.

In fact, experiment with all seven of our natural "tranquilizers." They give your nerves a chance to keep their cool under the heat of tension and stress, and are a healthy alternative to drugs. □

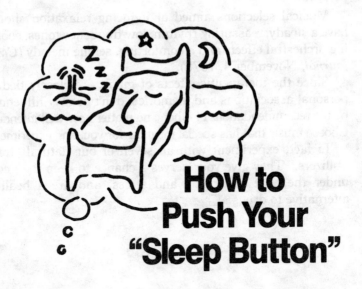

How to Push Your "Sleep Button"

Specialists are finding that simple relaxation techniques work better than sleeping pills.

Lying in bed, unable to fall asleep, is one of life's little tortures. Regrets about the past, tension in the present or anxiety about the future—these common aggravations can sometimes keep us up for hours. And almost all of us know the special frustration of losing sleep over the very task— an impending exam or job interview or long trip— that we need to be rested for.

For years, doctors casually prescribed sleeping pills for temporary insomnia. Many still do (to the tune of about 25 million prescriptions a year), but in the past several years, more and more physicians and psychologists are realizing that these drugs don't work and can be harmful if used frequently. A better way to send ourselves quickly to sleep, researchers are finding, is by learning simple skills—like muscle relaxation techniques, deep breathing, imagery, autogenic training and self-hypnosis—that can be applied when needed, without even leaving our beds.

Your body, as you lie there tossing and turning, is probably in a nightmarish state of biological turbulence. "Many poor sleepers are more aroused than good sleepers," writes sleep specialist Richard R. Bootzin, Ph.D., of Northwestern University, in a recent survey of sleep research. "Poor sleepers [have] higher rectal temperatures, higher skin resistance, more vasoconstrictions [narrowing of blood vessels] per minute and more body movements per hour than good sleepers." All of those symptoms mean that the insomniac's autonomic nervous system, which controls involuntary body functions, is preparing him perfectly for dodging rush-hour traffic—but not for sleep. If he can put his autonomic nervous system to sleep, the theory goes, the rest of him should follow (*Progress in Behavior Modification,* vol. 6, Academic Press, 1978).

Progressive relaxation is a particular form of muscle relaxation. Originated in the early 1900's by physiologist Edmund Jacobson, progressive relaxation or variations of it are still taught. One of these variations has been evaluated by Thomas D. Borkovec, Ph.D., a psychologist at Penn State University.

"We have the person start with the muscles of one hand, making a fist, holding it for seven seconds, and then relaxing it," says Dr. Borkovec, who teaches four-week and nine-week courses in relaxation.

"We ask the individual to learn to identify what both tension and relaxation feel like, so that he will be able to detect tension when trying to fall asleep. After sufficient practice, most people are able to deeply relax themselves within five minutes."

His students gradually learn to relax 16 of the body's muscle groups, Dr. Borkovec said. They also inhale when they tense their muscles, then exhale and relax very slowly (for about 45 seconds). That is good therapy for people whose main problem is falling asleep, and its effect improves with practice, Dr. Borkovec says.

Proper breathing, just by itself, is another way to reassure the autonomic nervous system that it can tone down for the night. In one experiment in 1976, volunteers were asked to "focus passively on the physical sensations associated with their breathing and to repeat the mantra [a word or image to fix the mind on] 'in' and 'out' silently." Results indicated that this technique is as effective as progressive relaxation.

'BREATHE THROUGH YOUR FINGERTIPS'

The fine points of breathing have been described by psychologist Beata Jencks, Ph.D., in her book, *Your Body: Biofeedback at Its Best* (Nelson-Hall, 1977).

"Imagine inhaling through your fingertips," Dr. Jencks writes, "up the arms, into the shoulders, and then exhaling down the trunk into the abdomen and legs, and leisurely out at the toes. Repeat, and feel how this slow, deep breathing affects the whole body, the abdomen, the flanks and the chest. Do not move the shoulders while doing the Long Breath."

To inhale deeply, Dr. Jencks advises, pretend to inhale the fragrance of the first flower in spring, or imagine that your breathing rises and falls like ocean waves, or that the surface area of your lungs—if laid out flat—would cover a tennis court. *That's* how much air you can feel youself breathing in.

Imagery can accompany breathing exercises, and your choice of images doesn't have to be limited to the traditional sheep leaping over a split-rail fence. Any image that you personally associate with feelings of peace or contentment will work well.

One sleep researcher, Quentin Regestein, M.D., director of the sleep clinic at Brigham and Women's Hospital in Boston, told us that one of his patients imagines a huge sculpture of the numeral one, hewn out of marble, with ivy growing over it, surrounded by a pleasant rural landscape. Then she goes on to the numeral two, and adds further embellishment, such as cherubs hovering above the numeral. "She tells me that she usually falls asleep before she reaches 50," Dr. Regestein says.

"Insomniacs come here from all over the world," he continues, "and ask me to prescribe a sleep cure for them. They are sometimes surprised to find that careful scientific investigation substantiates that commonsense remedies really work."

HEAVINESS AND WARMTH

Autogenic training is another natural and potent sleep aid. This technique acts on the premise that your mind can compel your body to relax by concentrating on feeling of heaviness and warmth. Through mental suggestion, the "heavy" muscles actually do relax, and the "warm" flesh receives better circulation, resulting in "a state of low physiological arousal," says Dr. Bootzin.

In an experiment in 1968, researchers taught 16 college-student insomniacs to focus their attention on warmth and heaviness. At the end of the experiment, the students had cut their average time needed to fall asleep down from 52 to 22 minutes. These results matched the findings made by Dr. Bootzin in the Chicago area in 1974: "Daily practice of either progressive relaxation or autogenic training produced 50 percent improvement in time to fall asleep by the end of the one-month treatment period."

A Raggedy Ann doll, says Dr. Jencks, is one image that can facilitate autogenic training. To feel heavy, she says, "make yourself comfortable and allow your eyes to close. Then lift one arm a little and let it drip. Let it drop heavily, as if it were the arm of one of those floppy dolls or animals. Choose one in your imagination. Choose a doll, an old, beloved, soft teddy bear." Once the mide fixes on the doll's image, Dr. Jencks says, lifting and dropping the arm in your imagination works as well as really letting it drop.

To invoke feelings of warmth, Dr. Jencks adds, "Imagine that you put your rag doll into the sun. Let it be warmed by the sun . . . . You are the giant rag doll, and you are lying in the sun; all your limbs are nice and warm, but your head is lying in the shade and is comfortably cool."

SUGGESTIONS YOU GIVE YOURSELF

Self-hypnosis, though it may require some practice in advance, has also been shown to help people fall asleep. Researchers in England compared the sleep-inducing ability of sleeping pills, hypnosis, self-hypnosis and a placebo on 18 volunteer insomniacs. Some of the volunteers learned to put themselves into a trance by picturing themselves in a "warm, safe place—possibly on a holiday someplace pleasant."

When they had put themselves into a trance, the researchers told them, they would be able to give themselves the suggestions "that this would pass into a deep, refreshing sleep, waking up at the usual time in the morning, feeling wide awake."

The results showed that the subjects fell asleep faster by hypnotizing themselves than by using either the drug or the placebo. None of the self-hypnotized sleepers needed an hour to fall asleep, while three in the placebo group and four in the drug group did. Twelve in the self-hypnotized group fell asleep in less than 30 minutes, while only seven and ten, respectively, in the other groups did (*Journal of the Royal Society of Medicine,* October, 1979).

Rituals also play a role in falling asleep. Dr. Regestein remarks that when dogs to to sleep, they always sniff around for a warm and comfortable spot, circle it, and finally coil up in their favorite sleeping position. People are a bit like this, he said. They fall asleep most easily when they proceed through a nightly ritual—flossing their teeth, for example, and then curling into their favorite sleeping position. In support of that theory, researchers in 1938 found that children who assumed a particular posture when going to bed, fell asleep faster.

The last, but not the least effective route to immediate relaxation is sexual activity. Psychologist Alice K. Schwartz, Ph.D., author of *Somniquest* (Harmony Books, 1979), a book dealing with sleep disturbances, says that sex "alleviates tension. It is a powerful soporific. And what is more, it's fun . . . The road to sleep branches into other byways. Explore all of them."

Finally, if none of the above techniques seem to work for you, there are several changes in daily habits that can, with practice, help you to fall asleep a lot faster in the future. Here are some hints that many sleep researchers recommend.

• Go to sleep and wake up at regular hours.
• Go to bed only when sleepy.
• Don't nap during the day.
• Use your bed only for sleeping and sex; don't read, eat or watch TV in bed.
• Keep your bedroom fairly cool.

If the inability to fall asleep becomes a chronic problem, the researchers suggest that you inspect other aspects of your life and behavior. Anything that can raise your blood pressure will keep you up. A constant state of tension over finances can do that; so can the habit of bottling up all kinds of emotions.

Two studies conducted by a team or researchers at the Penn State University Sleep Research and Treatment Center at Hershey, Pennsylvania, suggest that cigarette smoking is associated with insomnia and that quitting improves sleep within days after the last pack is thrown away (*Science,* February, 1980).

If, however, your lifestyle doesn't include any violations of those rules, any serious attempt to relax—by tensing and releasing the muscles, by deep breathing, by imagining yourself on a tropical isle, by self-hypnosis or by any mixture of the above—ought to soothe your autonomic nervous system and help you slip into restful sleep. □

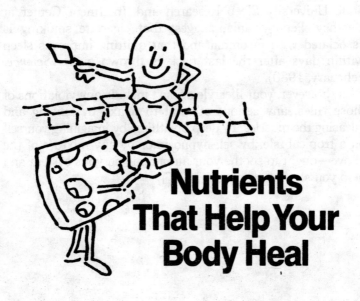

Nutrients That Help Your Body Heal

For fast, strong, infection-free wound healing, remember these crucial nutrients.

Imagine you were alive at the time of Homer's Greece, and in the heat of battle you caught a bronze-tipped arrow in the thigh. A valiant friend, carrying you on his back, managed to drag you off the battlefield and into the *klisia*, or medic's hut, before you passed out. What sort of first aid could you expect once you were there?

Well, if Homer's *Iliad* and *Odyssey* are any clues to ancient Grecian medical practice, you'd probably get: a seat, lots of storytelling, perhaps a cup of wine sprinkled with grated goat cheese and barley meal, served by a beautiful woman, and eventually, your wound would be washed out with warm water. To stanch the blood, you'd receive their most popular remedy—someone would recite a charm or sing a song over the injury. So much for the Red Cross.

Considering the amount of fighting the ancients did—and their crude if poetic ways of treating deadly wound—it's a wonder any of us are alive today. But (at least so far) the body's power of self-healing is greater than man's power of self-destruction. As one modern-day researcher has put it: "If the body were not wise, man could not survive. Every cell, tissue, organ and system is programmed to heal . . . The only reason we make it is that for every injury there is a healing response."

The healing of wounds is a process so intricate and marvelous that much of it remains a mystery today. But one thing is becoming increasingly certain: When your body is on the mend, whether it be from major surgery or a nicked knuckle, good nutrition can do a whole lot more to help it heal than telling it a story or singing it a song.

"I do believe that everyone should know the beautiful deeds of which his or her tissues are capable," writes Guido Majno, M.D., describing the physiological wonders of wound healing in his delightful book *The Healing Hand: Man and Wound in the Ancient World* (Harvard University Press, 1975). Those beautiful deeds include the ability to clean up the terrible mess caused by a wound, to fight off the invading hordes of bacteria, and to set about building brand-new tissues and blood vessels.

STEPPED-UP DEMAND

All this frantic activity at the site of the wound causes a stepped-up demand for carbohydrates, fats, minerals, vitamins, water, oxygen and — absolutely essential — amino acids, the famous building blocks of protein. And proteins are the bricks, boards and shingles of which the whole repair job is built.

In fact, "even more or less minor wounds require a good nutritional state and normal protein metabolism for optimal wound healing to take place," says Sheldon V. Pollack, M.D., chief of dermatologic surgery at Duke University Medical Center. Besides slowing down the reconstruction of tissues, protein deficiency can also impair the body's ability to protect itself from infection, Dr. Pollack observes. So when you're recovering from injury, it's doubly important to make sure your diet includes plenty of protein-rich foods, such as fish, milk, eggs, cheese, liver and wheat germ.

Injury also steps up the body's demand for certain nutrients, particularly vitamin C — a little hero of healing power.

Researchers have shown many times that "a deficiency of vitamin C impairs wound healing in experimental lower animals and human beings and . . . an excess accelerates healing above the normal level," write W.M. Ringsdorf Jr., D.M.D., and E. Cheraskin, M.D., of the University of Alabama School of Dentistry.

Vitamin C is a star in the cellular dramas of wound healing because it regulates the formation of collagen, a protein that's the main structural ingredient in connective tissue—the stuff your body uses to patch up its holes. When the cat nicks your hand, Dr. Majno explains, the wound is repaired "not with the original tissue but with a material that is biologically simple, cheap and handy: connective tissue . . . a soft but tough kind of tissue, specialized for mechanical functions, primarily that of holding us together; it fills the spaces in and around all other tissues."

Because the creation of collagen depends on vitamin C, a deficiency can disturb the "architecture" of that connective-tissue repair job, and delay the completion of the whole healing project. In one study, vitamin C deficiency in human cells decreased collagen production by 18 percent according to one biological measurement, and by 75 percent according to another measurement (*American Journal of Clinical Nutrition*, March, 1981.)

In another experiment, designed by Drs. Cheraskin and Ringsdorf, two gallant dental students with normal ascorbic acid (vitamin C) levels allowed the dentists to remove a tiny "plug" of tissue from their gums. In order to precisely measure the speed of healing, the wound was painted with a blue dye and photographed each day until the blue dot (indicating unhealed tissue) disappeared. After a two-week rest, the students had another "plug" extracted from their gums—but this time, they also took 250 milligrams of vitamin C with each meal and at bedtime (for a total of one gram daily).

A comparison of the healing sequences in both cases showed that the vitamin C-supplemented wounds healed 40 percent faster than those made when the students were eating a "normal" diet. When the experiment was repeated using a daily dose of two grams of vitamin C, the wounds healed 50 percent faster (*Oral Surgery, Oral Medicine, Oral Pathology,* March, 1982).

Actually, vitamin C's healing power has been recognized for decades. In the 1940's, A. H. Hunt reported that wound disruption or breakage had been reduced by 75 percent since doctors at St. Bartholomew's Hospital in London began routinely administering ascorbic acid to all patients having abdominal operations. Over a period of 30 months, Hunt observed that "leakage from suture lines has occurred in but one of a large number of operations."

More recently, in a British study, vitamin C's effect on the healing of bedsores was studied. Twenty surgical patients suffering from bedsores were divided into two groups: One group was given two 500 mg. vitamin C supplements daily, the other given two placebos (or chemically worthless pills). After a month, precise measurements of the wounds showed that the bedsores in the vitamin C group had decreased in size by 84 percent; the placebo group showed only a 42.7 percent decrease. "It is well established that in scurvy (vitamin C deficiency) wound healing is delayed and that the healing process may fail completely," the scientists observed (*Lancet,* September 7, 1974).

INJURY DRAINS VITAMIN C

When you're recovering from any kind of injury, it's also crucial to keep your diet vitamin C rich, because injury drains your body's supply. In one study, researchers found that ascorbic acid levels in the white blood cells of surgical patients had dropped by 42 percent three days after surgery (*Surgery, Gynecology and Obstetrics,* vol. 147, no. 1, 1978). Drs. Ringsdorf and Cheraskin suggest that this and other studies showing a drop in ascorbate levels may indicate that "during postsurgical recovery the vitamin C in the body migrates toward and concentrates in the healing site."

Whatever the case, Duke's Dr. Pollack told us, "If you're recovering from injury and you're seriously ill, elderly, don't eat properly or otherwise have low vitamin C levels, it would be wise to take one or two grams of vitamin C a day."

Zinc is another nutrient that has been widely studied as a possible accelerator of wound healing. Because it plays an important role in collagen formation, it seems logical that it would be involved in the body's "beautiful deeds" of healing—and a number of early studies caused excitement when it appeared that zinc really could speed up the healing process.

One study, for example, reported dramatic results in six patients on long-term corticosteroid therapy. Since chronic corticosteroid therapy is known to delay would healing, it came as something of a surprise that daily zinc supplementation resulted in the complete healing of all six patients' wounds (*Lancet,* April 14, 1973).

But later research produced conflicting results: Sometimes zinc worked, sometimes it didn't. One research team, after taking a look at the many studies of zinc and wound healing, pointed out that patients' serum zinc levels had not been measured before some of the studies were performed. "It is possible." they suggested, "that some of these patients receiving therapy with favorable results may have been zinc deficient prior to treatment" (*Journal of Surgical Research,* July, 1979).

Or, as another researcher put it, "supplemental zinc was indeed a stimulant to wound healing when administered to zinc-deficient individuals, but was of little value when given to those with an adequate zinc complement" (*Archives of Dermatology,* January, 1977).

In other words, if your zinc levels are normal, more zinc doesn't seem to help much; but if you're genuinely zinc deficient, it really can help.

Although the details of its role in wound healing aren't very well understood, vitamin A is known to be a player in collagen formation, wound closure and infection fighting. A plentiful supply of vitamin A can also help ensure that the new tissue that forms across the wound is strong and resistant to breaking, according to studies at the University of Illinois department of food science.

The Illinois investigators explored the effect of adding beta-carotene (a substance the body turns into vitamin A), and retinoic acid and retinyl acetate, two chemical forms of vitamin A, on the healing of wounds in rats with marginal vitamin A levels. The animals were fed a vitamin A-free diet for two weeks, then divided into groups: One received a "basal" diet, which provided a known amount of vitamin A, and the others received the basal diet plus one of the three vitamin A substances.

Five days later, when the animals were sacrificed and their

wounds examined, it was discovered that the supplemental retinyl acetate and beta-carotene "resulted in increases of 35 percent and 70 percent, respectively, over the wound tensile strength (resistance to being torn open) of rats fed the basal level of vitamin A" (*Federation Proceedings,* March 1, 1981, no. 3453).

Diabetics very often suffer from slow-healing wounds, a problem that can be worsened by another problem: They're also more apt to pick up an infection. But in a study conducted by researchers at the Albert Einstein College of Medicine, in New York City, supplemental vitamin A was shown to increase wound strength in diabetic animals. The researchers also believe that vitamin A helps fight wound infections.

The researchers concluded that vitamin A works to strengthen wounds mainly by increasing the accumulation of collagen. "We believe that just as supplemental vitamin A improves immune responses of traumatized animals and surgical patients, it will be especially useful in preventing wound infection and promoting wound healing in surgical diabetic patients," they observed (*Annals of Surgery,* July, 1981).

THIAMINE AND VITAMIN E: A LITTLE HELP FROM YOUR FRIENDS

There is also growing evidence that at least some of the B complex vitamins are involved in human wound healing. In one recent study, experimental animals fed diets rich in thiamine (vitamin B1) were found to have heavier, denser granulation tissue (new tissue formed during wound repair) than those on deficient diets.

Based on thiamine's known biological activities in the body, the researchers concluded it probably aids healing by helping the body step up its energy metabolism at the healing site, where the furious breakdown and buildup of cells requires tremendous amounts of usable fuel (*Journal of Surgical Research,* January, 1982).

But no survey of nutrition and wound healing would be complete without mention of vitamin E.

Wilfrid E. Shute, M.D., a veteran vitamin E researcher, reported that vitamin E helps accelerate wound healing, is "the ideal treatment for burns" because of its ability to limit cell death to those cells that have been killed by the burning agent, and can even help reduce old scar tissue when applied directly. Keloids, or progressively enlarging, raised scars caused by overproduction of collagen during the healing process, can be prevented by taking vitamin E orally and also applying it directly to the fresh wound, Dr. Shute says.

Not everyone agrees. Dr. Pollack, while observing that "there is some data to suggest that vitamin E can promote wound healing," told us that "the research is still kind of up in the air . . . we just don't know the precise role, if any, that vitamin E plays in wound healing."

But meanwhile, next time you peel your knuckle along with the potato — or catch a Grecian arrow in the thigh — you might give nutrition a try. It could just be your body knows some things your doctor doesn't. □

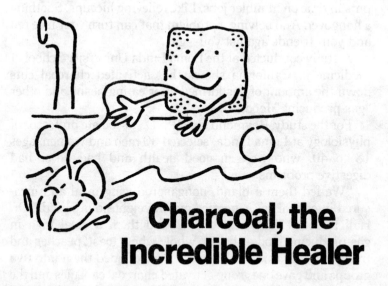

Charcoal, the Incredible Healer

Using an 'activated' form of this natural product, doctors are treating everything from gas and intestinal ailments to serious infections.

The year is 1813, and the French chemist Claude Bertrand is in his laboratory, a vial in his hand. It contains a teaspoonful of arsenic, enough to kill 150 men. He lifts it to his lips, swallows it—and goes about his business as if nothing had happened. And nothing had.

Bertrand wasn't committing suicide, he was conducting an experiment. One he lived to tell about. He survived because the arsenic was mixed with *charcoal,* a substance that acted like a sponge in his stomach and sucked up the arsenic before it reached his blood. A century later, charcoal filters in gas masks protected World War I soldiers from poison gas. And today, charcoal—made more effective by a process called "activation"—is used in submarines and space capsules to purify the air. It's also used in emergency rooms to treat victims of poisoning or drug overdose.

But activated charcoal is more than a lifesaving hero. It also puts in time on humbler jobs. Like relieving hiccups. Soothing a hangover. And solving a problem that can turn your face red and your friends against you — gas.

A study conducted at the Loma Linda University School of Medicine in California shows that activated charcoal cuts down the amount of gas formed after eating beans and other "gas-producing" foods.

For the study, Raymond Hall, Ph.D., associate professor of physiology at Loma Linda, selected 30 men and women, ages 18 to 40, who were in good health and had never had digestive problems.

"We fed them a bland, nongasproducing meal and measured intestinal gas generated over an eight-hour period," Dr. Hall told us. "The next day we fed them a meal high in gas-producing foods — beans, whole wheat toast, peaches and fruit juice. For this meal, however, we divided them into two groups and gave one group activated charcoal capsules and the other placebos (identical looking pills with nothing of value)."

The group receiving placebos, says Dr. Hall, produced large amounts of gas. But the group receiving activated charcoal produced much less — *no more, in fact, than after the bland meal.* And when the two groups ate another gassy meal, this time with the placebo group receiving the activated charcoal and vice versa, the results repeated themselves: placebo group, lots of gas; activated charcoal group, gas levels same as the bland meal.

"Activated charcoal reduced the amount of gas either by absorbing the gas itself or absorbing the intestinal bacteria that produce the gas," explains Dr. Hall.

But no matter how it works, Dr. Hall believes activated charcoal is "a good cure for gas. If a person has a gas problem, it's well worth trying."

For best results, Dr. Hall suggests taking activated charcoal shortly after a meal. But, he emphasizes, activated charcoal won't quickly clear up a case of gas that's already developed. "It takes several hours for activated charcoal to reach the lower intestinal tract where the gas is being produced," he says.

GOOD FOR 'TURISTA'

Since activated charcoal stifles bacteria in the intestines, Dr. Hall believes it may also cure mild dysentery—better known as "turista."

Sharing that opinion is Marjorie Baldwin, M.D., a doctor at the Wildwood Sanitarium and Hospital in Wildwood, Georgia. "Charcoal is an excellent remedy for traveler's diarrhea," she told us.

But Dr. Baldwin uses activated charcoal for more than just gas and diarrhea. "Any inflammation—an area that is red, painful, swollen and hot—responds to charcoal. We apply charcoal as a poultice if the inflammation is on the outside of the body or give it by mouth if the inflammation is in the digestive tract."

Dr. Baldwin describes the case of a juvenile diabetic whose foot was saved from amputation by charcoal.

"This young lady had caught pneumonia and her feet were soaked in hot water. Because she was diabetic, her feet were damaged and she developed severe infections. Antibiotics didn't clear them up. The doctors suggested one foot be amputated, but she refused and came to us for treatment. We put that foot in a plastic bag filled with a mixture of charcoal and water that was about the consistency of cream. The foot was kept in the bag round the clock, and the mixture was changed four times a day. She walked out of our clinic—on both feet."

Doctors in England have also used charcoal to treat infections. A letter to *Lancet* (September 13, 1980), one of the world's most prestigious medical journals, describes the use of charcoal-saturated cloth for wounds that were infected, discharging and had a bad odor.

The doctors applied a single layer of the charcoal cloth to the wounds of 26 patients with chronic leg ulcers and 13 patients with unhealed surgical incisions. "A noticeable reduction in wound odor occurred in 24 ulcer patients and 13 surgical wound patients," the doctors write. And they found the charcoal cloth reduced odor longer than "standard dressing materials."

The doctors note that charcoal may have reduced the odor by absorbing bacteria. It's a possible explanation since, says

Dr. Baldwin, "charcoal is the most powerful absorbent known to man.

"Charcoal absorbs up to thousands of times its own weight," she explains. "It has enormous surface area—like a football field-sized piece of tissue paper rolled up into a tiny ball—and the more surface area charcoal has, the more absorbent it is." (One pound of activated charcoal has a surface area equal to 125 acres!)

EFFECTIVE FIRST AID

And charcoal absorbs poisons. So effectively, that it's an ingredient in the "universal antidote," a concoction designed to take on almost any poison known to man. But even by itself, charcoal tackles a wide array or poisons—from hemlock to DDT. That versatility prompted a pair of Army doctors, writing in the medical journal *Pediatrics* (September, 1974), to recommend that every family keep activated charcoal on hand to deal with poisoning emergencies.

"It is immediately effective upon ingestion and can be given safely by nonprofessionals," they write. "Hence, its inclusion in household first aid supplies is warranted." (To neutralize poison, mix about one-quarter to one-half cup powdered charcoal with a cup of water, stir or shake the mixture, and have the victim drink it within the first 30 minutes after the poisoning. And, of course, go to a doctor, poison center or emergency room.)

And if you pick your "poison" one too many times, charcoal may be the best antidote for a hangover.

Hangovers are caused by substances called congeners—and activated charcoal absorbs them. In an experiment conducted at Columbia University College of Pharmaceutical Sciences in New York City, researchers found that in test-tube conditions similar to a person's stomach, activated charcoal absorbed 93 percent of one congener and 82 percent of another.

HANGOVER HELP

In a second experiment, 68 volunteers—nondrinkers and moderate social drinkers—drank either two ounces of whiskey, which has a high level of congeners, or two ounces of charcoal-filtered vodka, which has almost none. The researchers then measured their hangover symptoms the next day.

Twenty-five percent of the whiskey group had stomach-aches, 27 percent had bad breath, nine percent had head-aches, seven percent had dizziness and six percent had fatigue. On the other hand, only two percent of the vodka groups had headaches or stomach upset, and there was no bad breath, dizziness or fatigue (*Southwestern Medicine,* September, 1971).

Charcoal may also solve another problem—hiccups.

"I have treated my cases of hiccups with charcoal tablets," wrote a doctor to the *British Medical Journal* (September 10, 1977), "and have instructed patients to continue chewing them at least once an hour and in extreme cases continuously. In most cases I have met with success on this simple regimen."

On a more sober note, doctors use activated charcoal to treat patients with kidney failure. Those patients often have high levels of blood fats (arteriosclerosis is the leading cause of death in patients on long-term hemodialysis, the treatment for kidney patients that mechanically cleans their blood).

And they often suffer from severe itching.

If you have high cholesterol, or an itch that doesn't quit, should you take activated charcoal regularly?

No.

"I wouldn't recommend activated charcoal as a daily supplement," says Dr. Baldwin.

Charcoal, she explains, "doesn't know what's naughty and what's not," and absorbs vitamins along with any bad substances. And although no one who has taken activated charcoal has been known to develop a vitamin deficiency—or any other health problem from the charcoal—Dr. Baldwin believes it's best used selectively.

"Charcoal takes toxins out of the system so the body can get well," she says. "For gas, diarrhea, infections and poisonings—charcoal works." □

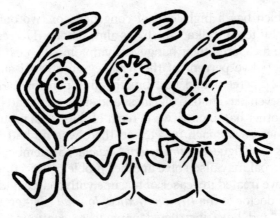

Plant Your Own Outdoor Medicine Chest

*Eight easy-to-grow medicinal herbs
treasured for soothing relief of minor ailments.*

Almost everyone is gardening these days. What with food prices so high and no end in sight, there's hardly a family around that hasn't plowed up at least part of the backyard to grow a variety of vegetables and fruits.

Now, however, another kind of crop is starting to take up residence in neighborhoods all over America—bushy, aromatic herbs.

We all know there's nothing like herbs to add flavor and spice to everyday foods. But thousands of years ago, it was their medicinal properties that made them so valuable. They were the "wonder drugs" of the Romans, Egyptians, Europeans and others who developed comprehensive herbal remedies.

Too bad most of them have been lost in the rush for today's modern miracle cures, because there's still plenty to say in favor of those old-time practices. Whether it's an herb tea to soothe a sore throat and loosen a cough or a poultice of herbs to lessen the pain of arthritis or sprains, there's a place for that kind of treatment in every home.

So while you're growing your vegetables this summer, why not add some herbs to the family plot? You can start some of them from seed or you can buy plants from a nursery for use this summer. And we'll tell you how to get others started from seeds or cuttings so you'll be all set for *next* spring, or maybe even for a little indoor gardening during the off season.

We've compiled a list of eight practical medicinal herbs you can grow yourself, although there are lots more. Some of them you'll recognize immediately because of their popularity as seasonings. But all of them, whether you know it or not, have properties that also classify them as medicinal.

HERBS AREN'T FUSSY

Best of all, herbs practically raise themselves. Most like an open, sunny, well-drained spot, somewhat sheltered from the wind. But the soil need not be rich; in fact, it's actually better in some cases if it isn't. And herbs are seldom bothered to any extent by bugs.

All of the herbs we're discussing are perennials, which means they'll come up year after year. The plant itself may be killed by the frost, but the roots hibernating all winter will send up new shoots at the crack of spring.

Still, some herbs are more tender than others. So it's a good idea not to plant outdoors until all danger of frost is past.

You can begin harvesting your herbs much sooner than you might think. The leaves of an herb plant can be picked at almost any time, though peak flavor is reached just before flowering. Picking stimulates new growth—so don't hold back. In fact, you can pull off up to a third of the plant all at once without doing any harm.

Once you've got the leaves, you can use them fresh or preserve them for the future by drying them. The same can be done with flowers and seedheads, too.

To dry, arrange the herbs (leaves, seeds or flowers) in thin layers on clean paper, cookie sheets or best of all, screens or mesh. Allow to air-dry. They'll take two days to two weeks to become brittle. Store in airtight glass jars in a dark place away from excessive heat.

Herbs can also be hung in bunches to dry, or you can dry them in your kitchen oven. But you must be careful not to overheat, or the aromatic oils will evaporate.

Dried leaves are more concentrated than fresh, so recipes will have to be adjusted to compensate for that. For example, when making an herb tea, put in one teaspoon per cup if you are using dried herbs and two if fresh.

"Some herb teas are best when made with fresh leaves, but you can use dried, too." says Bonnie Fisher, author of *Bonnie Fisher's Way With Herbs Cookbook* (Keats, 1980). Mrs. Fisher has been growing herbs for years. "Once I got started, I couldn't stop," she says. "The first year I planted only basil. Then I got curious and started reading books on the subject and experimenting on my own. Now I grow 125 different herbs. Interest is really catching on. Eight or so years ago it was almost impossible to find herb seeds, let alone plants. Now it's much easier to get what you need."

Of course, our list of medicinal herbs isn't a complete one. That would take volumes. Our group is intended to pique your interest and help you get started with your own herb garden, whether you're a seasoned gardener or a novice.

SAGE

Common sage is an attractive shrubby perennial growing from 18 inches to two feet. It has gray-green pebble-textured leaves and clusters of lilac-blue flowers. Sage is readily propagated from seed—you can start it outdoors after the last frost. The plants will grow in any kind of soil if they have full sun. Take care not to water from above in the evening, as sage can develop mildew from that practice.

Use the leaves from the matured plant either fresh or dried.

Sage is valued for counteracting rich and greasy foods such as goose and duck. That's probably why it has a reputation to this day as a digestive aid. In fact, many who take sage for intestinal inflammation testify that the strong, camphorous, slightly bitter tea is quite effective.

But that's not all it's used for. Some gargle with sage tea to relieve sore throat or bleeding gums. And the tea, made extra strong, is an excellent lotion for raw abrasions of the skin.

HORSERADISH

This sassy herb is best propagated from root cuttings. The cuttings should be about eight or nine inches long and have a crown or growing point. Plant 12 to 15 inches deep in soil that is rich, moist and well supplied with organic matter. Except for clearing the weeds, no further care is needed.

Horseradish is a vigorous perennial that can easily get out of hand. For that reason you may want to give it private room for growing.

The plant itself can reach a height of two feet and be about as wide. But it's only the root that is used for food or medicine. The root can be stored in a cool cellar, barn, outdoor pit or cold storage and will keep for months.

To use, just grate some of the fresh raw root. You'll immediately notice its pungent odor and hot, biting taste.

When eaten, horseradish acts as a potent diuretic. In fact it's the diuretic properties that make horseradish useful for gout and rheumatic problems and for bladder infections.

Externally, horseradish is used as an irritant to stimulate blood flow. It can also be made into a poultice for rheumatism.

Horseradish juice mixed with white vinegar is said to help remove freckles when applied to the skin.

GARLIC

Growing garlic is almost foolproof. The soil may be sandy, loam or clay, but garlic grows best in a rich, moist, sandy soil. Just divide the garlic bulb into its component cloves and plant them in a sunny spot about two inches deep and about six inches apart, leaving about a foot between rows. And keep them free from weeds.

The bulbs should be ready to harvest when the leaves of the plant turn brown and dry. In the off season, you can plant the cloves in a pot placed on a sunny windowsill.

Everyone knows how garlic enhances the flavor of foods. But you'll be glad to know that scientists have confirmed that garlic stimulates the flow of gastric juices and aids digestion. It dilates blood vessels and has been used successfully to relieve high blood pressure.

ROSEMARY

Rosemary is a sun-loving evergreen that flourished best in poor, sandy, well-drained and limes soils. It's a tender perennial, which means it may not make it through a harsh winter. For that reason, rosemary is ideal for growing indoors in a pot about 10 inches in diameter. Outdoors it will grow to as much as five feet, but indoors this bushy, needlelike evergreen can be kept to a reasonable height of about two feet by pinching back or harvesting tip cuttings.

"Either way, this is one herb you probably will not want to start from seed," says Bonnie Fisher, "unless you're very patient. Seeds generally take three to four weeks to germinate, if at all. You're better off getting plants or cuttings." Place them about three feet apart outdoors or one to a pot indoors. But no matter where it is grown, rosemary must never be allowed to dry out or be subjected to temperatures below 27°.

The leaves are used either fresh or dried. Use as a seasoning, but try it as a tea, too. In that form, it's been prescribed for everything from bad breath (it has a piney taste) to hair loss. In fact, it's still an ingredient in hair oils. Rosemary is believed to cure headaches, strengthen the memory, stimulate the appetite and quiet coughs. The tea has even been used externally to clear the complexion.

CAMOMILE

Camomile is a low-growing, apple-scented, matlike perennial whose flowers are remarkably daisylike.

In fact, it's the flowers that are most often used for medicinal purposes. Maude Grieve says a camomile tea made by mixing one ounce of the flowers to a pint of boiling water has a wonderfully soothing, sedative effect. It's considered a preventive for nightmares and has sometimes been employed in intermittent fevers.

Camomile flowers are also used as a poultice for external swelling, inflammatory pain, earache and toothache. It's even used to relieve the problem of sore gums.

"For months I had been enduring discomfort and pain resulting from irritated and inflamed gums," another letter writer told us. "I went to a dentist, and he suggested I have two teeth pulled. My 'gut feeling' told me that my teeth did not have to be pulled!

"Instinctively, I tried rinsing my mouth with luke warm camomile tea. You cannot imagine what relief that brought! It was like a soothing, calming effect that 'put out the fire' that had seemed to be burning my gums. I continue to rinse with camomile tea after each brushing."

Camomile can be started from seed in well-drained, rather dry, sandy soil. Thin the seedlings so they are about 18 inches apart. They should be pressed in firmly and kept well weeded. Once established they'll produce runners, which should be divided the following spring for further plant propagation.

Or purchase some mature, double-flowered plants to begin with. Camomile doesn't require especially fertile soil, but add cow manure to insure an adequate supply of nitrogen.

The herb stays low except while in bloom. The foliage is very fine and fernlike with a delicate sprinkling of white flowers, almost too pretty to pick.

PEPPERMINT

Mints will grow almost anywhere, but thrive in moist, rich soil in shade or sun. Peppermint is best started by cuttings or root divisions of a bought plant and grows to about four feet tall. It has small reddish-violet flowers, which along with the leaves give off the characteristic menthol aroma when crushed.

Mint grows from creeping roots and spreads so rapidly that it can wreak havoc in your herb garden. For that reason you may want to plant it in a bed by itself in a big tub or indoors in a pot. Actually, you probably won't mind that it grows so prolifically because there are so many uses for this herb.

Brew a tea of peppermint to alleviate nausea, flatulence and colic. It's also good for raising internal heat and inducing perspiration. It can be taken for nervousness, insomnia, poor digestion, heartburn and migraine headaches.

"In slight colds or early indications of disease," claims Maude Grieve, "A free use of peppermint tea will, in most cases, effect a cure."

Made into a salve or a bath additive, it can relieve itching skin conditions.

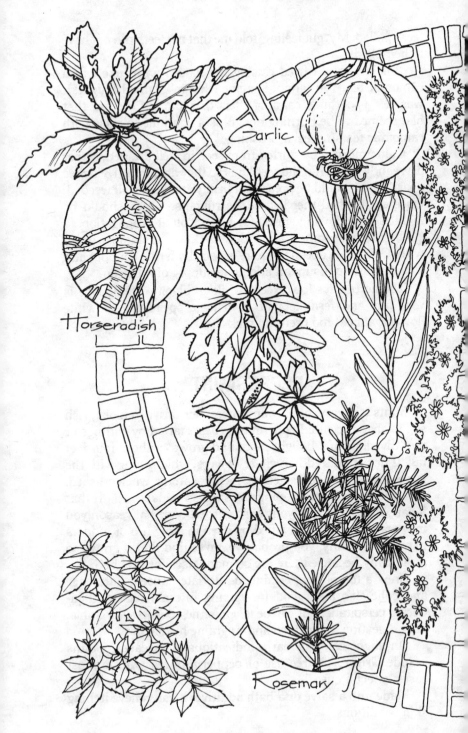

Garlic

Horseradish

Rosemary

64

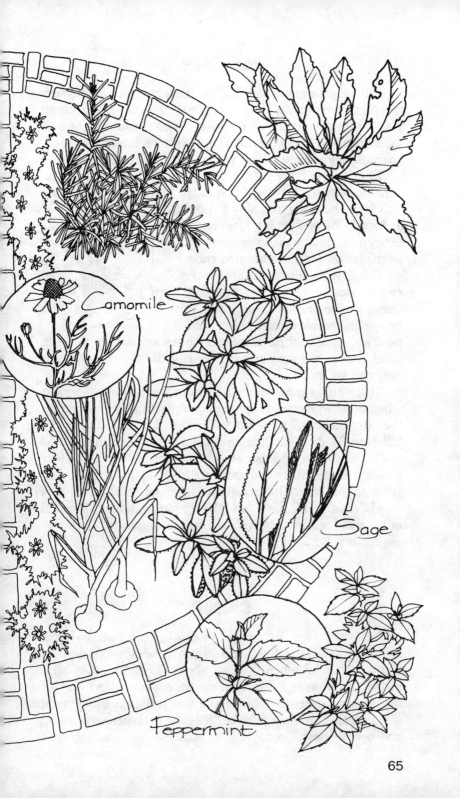

Camomile

Sage

Peppermint

65

PLANTAIN

You may be more familiar with plantain as a common perennial weed than as a medicinal herb. That's because plantain grows profusely on lawns, along roadsides and in meadowlands. It can overtake your lawn if allowed to spread, so think twice about where you want to sow seeds.

You can recognize plantain by its oval, smooth, thickish leaves, which range from 4 to 10 inches long and about two-thirds as broad. Purplish-green flowers, held on long erect stalks, reach the same length as the leaves but have blunted ends.

The flowers, along with the leaves, can be used to treat any number of minor problems. The fresh leaves can be applied whole or bruised in the form of a poultice, then rubbed over insect bites and stings to bring relief from pain. Plantain may even stop the bleeding of minor cuts and scrapes.

"The itching associated with poison ivy can be . . . stopped when crushed leaves of the common plantain are rubbed on the affected area," says Serge Duckett, M.D., Ph.D., of the Jefferson Medical College in Philadelphia. And he should know, because he had success with it himself. So pleased was he with the results that he had since treated 10 others afflicted with poison ivy. "The cessation of itching in all cases was rapid," says Dr. Duckett, "and the dermatitis did not spread to other areas of the body" (*New England Journal of Medicine,* September 4, 1980).

CATNIP

As its name implies, cats adore this herb and will go into a state of ecstatic abandon over it. "Even mountain lions become silly and playful when they get ahold of catnip," says Mrs. Fisher. On humans, however, it has the opposite effect, and for that reason catnip tea (which has a minty, slightly bitter taste) is often used as a sleep inducer. "It's good in restlessness, colic, and nervousness," according to Maude Grieve, author of *A*

Modern Herbal (Dover Publications, 1971). She also says that catnip will relieve painful swellings when it is applied in the form of a poultice.

A woman from Cameron, Missouri, found yet another use for catnip. "I suffered with a stomach ulcer for several years, trying all sort of remedies," she told us in a letter. "Finally, I tried catnip tea. It worked like a charm; my ulcer was gone in practically no time."

Whether you use catnip as a tea or a poultice, you'll find that it is quite easy to grow as long as you have well-drained soil. It can be started from seeds, plants or stem cuttings.

In the spring it's pretty easy to use cuttings; stem ends four inches long stuck into soil or other planting media will usually root within a week.

Harvest the catnip when half the blossoms are open, early in the day after the dew has evaporated.

For medicinal purposes use two or three heaping teaspoons of catnip in a cup of boiling water. Steep for 10 minutes. Add honey and drink your catnip tea as you like it—hot or cold.

A WORD ABOUT SAFETY

A few words of caution. Never take any herb internally (or, externally for that matter) unless you know exactly what it is and what it may do. Even so-called safe ones may cause some upset if taken too freely.

We don't recommend herbs in pill form, either. Stick to weak herbal teas or culinary herbs. Most of all, don't forget to take the time to enjoy your garden. "In the cool of early morning," says Adelma Simmons, author of *Herb Gardening in Five Seasons* (Hawthorn Books, 1964), "evaluate your plants and appreciate their beauty. Brush fragrant plants, roll a leaf or two in your hand, and breath in the wonderful aroma. □

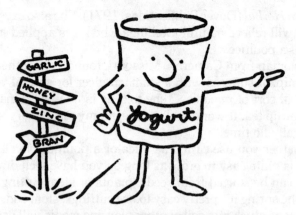

Quick Guide to Stocking Your Natural Medicine Cabinet

☐ GARLIC

reduces nasal congestion;
reported to reduce cholesterol levels;
relieves gas, aids digestion

☐ BREWER'S YEAST

provides essential B vitamins and chromium;
helps to combat stress

☐ HONEY

used topically to aid dry skin;
used in tea to soothe sore throat

☐ BRAN

relieves constipation by providing bulk;
may protect body from hemorrhoids and diverticular disease

☐ ALOE VERA

used topically to soothe and assist healing of minor burns and
wounds and other minor skin irritations

☐ VITAMIN C

thought to increase resistance to infectious diseases;
believed to decrease duration of colds;
may accelerate wound healing

☐ VITAMIN E

used topically to provide relief from minor skin irritations,
cuts, burns and rashes such as poison ivy

☐ VITAMIN A

helps body fight infection

☐ CHARCOAL

helps to prevent gas, alleviate diarrhea, hangovers, intestinal
infections

☐ ZINC

thought to help clear up acne, fight infection and heal wounds

☐ YOGURT (with live bacteria)

can help sooth cold sores;
helps promote healthy intestines;
used topically to help heal vaginal infections ☐

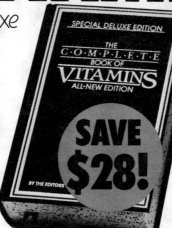

Rodale Press, Inc., publishes PREVENTION,® the better health magazine.
For information on how to order your subscription,
write to PREVENTION,® Emmaus, PA 18049.